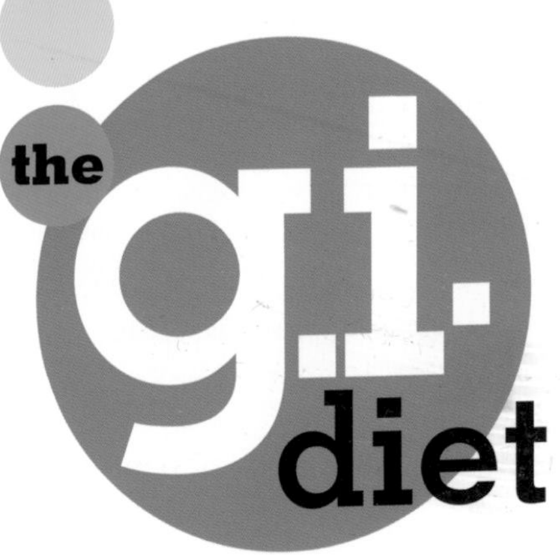

GUIDE TO SHOPPING AND EATING OUT

RICK GALLOP

Past President of the Heart and Stroke Foundation of Ontario

RANDOM HOUSE CANADA

 Published in 2010 by Random House Canada, a division of Random House of Canada Limited. Distributed in Canada by Random House of Canada Limited.

www.randomhouse.ca

Library and Archives Canada Cataloguing in Publication

Gallop, Rick
The revised G.I. diet guide to shopping and eating out / Rick Gallop.

Includes index.
ISBN 978-0-307-35833-2

1. Glycemic index. 2. Reducing diets. I. Title.
RM222.2.G3427 2009 613.2'5 C2009-904344-0

Printed and bound in Canada

10 9 8 7 6 5 4 3 2 1

Contents

Introduction

Congratulations! The fact that you're reading this means you've decided to go on the G.I. Diet—the easiest, healthiest, most effective route to permanent weight loss. Whether you've been losing weight on the plan for a while or are just about to embark on it, *The Revised G.I. Diet Guide to Shopping and Eating Out* is a convenient pocket guide that will not only make following the program easier, but will show you how much fun you can have while losing weight. Being on the G.I. Diet doesn't mean you have to radically change your lifestyle. It was designed with the real world in mind so that you can dine out, travel, celebrate special events, snack and still lose those extra unwanted pounds. No matter where you go or what the occasion, there are always delicious green-light options to enjoy, and the purpose of this book is to list them for you.

It's intended to be a complementary tool with The G.I. Diet series of books, and not a replacement for them, since it doesn't explain the principles of the diet or how it works. Rather it's to be carried and consulted on your weekly grocery trip, as you grab a bite on the run or when you're out with friends at your favourite restaurant.

This book is divided into two main sections. Part One, "At the Grocery Store," takes you aisle by aisle through the supermarket. While the food guides in The G.I. Diet series are organized by meal or food group, this guide is organized the way a typical grocery store is, starting with the produce section and ending with frozen foods. You can start at the beginning and let the book navigate your shopping cart through the supermarket aisles, or you can look up a specific food in the index, which starts on page 93.

Part Two, "Eating Out," lists the green-light options available at a number of popular fast food chains and also gives some helpful guidelines to follow while dining out. It lists the dishes you'd typically find at Italian, Greek, Chinese, Indian, Mexican, Thai and Japanese restaurants and points out the green-light options. Eating out should be a fun social occasion and this guide will help you enjoy it without worrying about your waistline.

One of the most popular features of the G.I. Diet is that you don't have to count calories, add points or measure carbs in order to follow it. I've been researching glycemic ratings, fat and calorie levels, and ingredient lists of food products and menu items, and have done all the math for you. Now all you have to do is look at the colour-coded charts to find out which foods you can fill your shopping cart with or order in a restaurant. Although I've included the red- and yellow-light columns along with the green-light, this book is really about the green-light, about all the foods you can enjoy while slimming down. This diet isn't about deprivation and going hungry, it's about making the right choices and eating until you're satisfied. Food is one of life's greatest pleasures and you can definitely indulge in it. Enjoy!

As always, your feedback is extremely valuable. I can be reached through my website, at **www.gidiet.com.**

PART ONE

At the Grocery Store

The Green-Light Grocery Guide

Following the G.I. Diet really begins once you clear out your pantry and refrigerator of red-light products and make a trip to the grocery store to stock up on green-light ones. A word of advice: don't go to the supermarket until after you've eaten a meal. One of the worst mistakes you can make is to go grocery shopping on an empty stomach—you'll only feel tempted by all those red-light ready-to-eat foods. You may also want to do a bit of planning before you go. Check out the recipe sections in the G.I. Diet books, especially *The G.I. Diet Cookbook*, choose a few that appeal to you and make a list of the ingredients you'll need. Then take it and this guide along with you to the store. With these tools in hand, you'll find it easy to load your cart with delicious food, and I hope you'll be introduced to some new favourites.

HOW TO USE THIS GUIDE

I've organized the food in this guide the way you would typically find it in the supermarket, in sections such as the Produce Aisle, the Deli Counter, the Bakery, the Meat Counter, the Beverage Aisle, the Frozen Food Section and so on. Within each of these sections, you'll find categories of food such as vegetables, processed meat, breads, etc. All are listed in one of the three traffic-light-based colour columns.

If you find a food in the red-light column that you would normally add to your shopping cart, look at what's listed beside it in the green-light column. There is almost always a wonderful green-light alternative to a red- or yellow-light food. If, for example, you would normally buy a cantaloupe, which is a red-light food, choose some peaches or oranges or grapes, or any of the other green-light choices instead. Remember that if you want to look up a specific food rather than a whole category, you can look at the index on pages 93–101.

I've generally tried to stay away from listing specific brands. There are just far too many out there and they vary from region to region. For the most part they don't have any bearing on the G.I. rating of a particular food anyway. For example, 1% cottage cheese or whole wheat spaghetti or Dijon mustard is pretty much the same no matter who's made it. The only times I have mentioned brands is when it does make a difference. For example, most cold cereals are red light, but Kashi Go Lean is a green-light product.

It can be a bit tricky sometimes trying to distinguish the green-light products from the red-light. Take bread for example. We know that white bread is red-light, since it spikes glucose levels in your bloodstream, releasing insulin, which stores the glucose as fat. The green-light alternative is whole-grain bread, but many of the healthy-looking multi-grain loaves out there are not exactly what they seem. Some of them list "enriched white flour" or "unbleached flour" in the ingredient list, and this puts a red flashing light over them. The first ingredient listed on bread should always be "100% whole wheat flour" or "100% whole-grain flour." If "stone-ground" is mentioned, even better. So checking ingredient lists and labels can be important, and I'll give you some guidelines to follow.

READING LABELS

When buying a green-light food such as a loaf of whole wheat bread or a bottle of low-fat salad dressing, you'll find several kinds to choose from. How do you decide which to add to your shopping cart? Read the nutritional label on the package. Now, I know these labels aren't exactly consumer friendly, but they do contain some helpful information. Here are the seven key components that will help you make the best choice:

1. **Serving size:** Is this realistic, or is the manufacturer low-balling it so the calorie and fat content look better than the competition? When comparing one brand with another, make sure you're comparing the same serving sizes.

2. **Calories:** The product with the least amount of calories is obviously the best choice.

3. **Fat:** Choose the product with the least amount of fat, particularly saturated fat, and avoid any product that contains trans fat—the worst of the saturated fats.

4. Protein: The higher the protein level, the better. Protein acts as a brake on the digestive system, lowering the G.I. rating of the food.

5. Fibre: The product with the higher fibre content is the best choice, whether it's soluble or insoluble. Fibre, like protein, significantly lowers the G.I. rating.

6. Sugar: Try to avoid products that contain added sugar. Choose the ones with sugar substitutes or none at all. "Nonfat" products that contain added sugar aren't non-fattening!

7. Sodium (Salt): Look for lower sodium levels. Sodium increases water retention, which causes bloating and added weight and impacts blood pressure.

Nutrition Facts	
Serving Size 1 cup (236ml)	
Servings Per Container 1	
Amount Per Serving	
Calories 80	Calories from Fat 0
	% Daily Value*
Total Fat 0g	**0%**
Saturated Fat 0g	**0%**
Trans Fat 0g	
Cholesterol Less than 5mg	**0%**
Sodium 120mg	**5%**
Total Carbohydtrate 11g	**4%**
Dietary Fiber 0g	**0%**
Sugars 11g	
Protien 9g	**17%**
Vitamin A 10% •	Vitamin C 4%
Calcium 30% • Iron 0% • Vitamin D 25%	

* Percent Daily Values are based on a 2,000 calorie diet. Your daily values may be higher or lower depending on your calorie needs.

Serving Size: make sure you are comparing the same serving size

Calories: pick the lower calorie level

Fat: the lower the fat, especially saturated fat, the better

Salt: generally, the less the better

Fiber: higher is best, as it helps reduce the G.I.

Sugar: low, low, low

Protein: higher is better—protein helps slow digestion

TO SUM UP

The best green-light buy is

- Lower in calories
- Lower in fat, particularly saturated fat
- Higher in fibre
- Lower in sugar and sodium.

THE PRODUCE AISLE

Vegetables and fruit are the cornerstone of the G.I. Diet. They are low G.I. and high in fibre, nutrients, vitamins and minerals. Cooking them raises their G.I. and reduces their nutrient content, so microwave or steam vegetables using as little water as possible and cook only until they are crisp-tender—or try eating them raw.

Frozen fruits and vegetables are just as nutritious as fresh. They also taste great as they are picked at precisely the right time. Large family size packs are relatively inexpensive and have the advantage of being available year-round.

Soy-based foods such as tofu are high in protein, low in saturated fat and good for a healthy heart. Many supermarkets carry something called veggie ground round, which looks and tastes exactly like ground beef, but is made of Textured Vegetable Protein (TVP). TVP is used to make veggie burgers, veggie breakfast links and other products. It's an excellent choice whether you're vegetarian or not.

You can often find nuts and dried fruit in the produce section of the supermarket. Most dried fruit is very high in sugar and therefore red-light. However there are some yellow-light choices, and all dried fruit can be used in modest quantities in baking.

Nuts are an excellent source of good fats and protein, and green-light nuts contain even more monounsaturated (best) fat than the others. Remember, though, that all nuts are calorie dense and so must be eaten in limited quantities, about eight to twelve per serving. It's just too easy to unconsciously consume a whole bowl of nuts while watching television, but this quantity would equal your total calorie needs for an entire day!

VEGETABLES

Broad Beans	Artichokes	Alfalfa sprouts
Coleslaw (commercial)	Beets	Arugula
Parsnips	Corn	Asparagus
Plantains	Potatoes (boiled)	Beans (green/wax)
Potatoes (mashed, baked, fried)	Pumpkin	Belgian endive
Rutabaga	Squash	Bell peppers
Turnip	Sweet potatoes	Bok choy
	Yams	Broccoli
		Brussels sprouts
		Cabbage (all varieties)
		Carrots
		Cauliflower

VEGETABLES

		Celery Celery root Collard greens Cucumbers Edamame (soy beans) Eggplant Escarole Fennel Fiddleheads Fresh herbs Garlic Gingerroot Green onions Horseradish Kale Kohlrabi Leeks Lettuce (all varieties) Mushrooms (all varieties) Mustard greens Potatoes (small, preferably new) Okra Onions

VEGETABLES		
		Peas Peppers (sweet or hot) Radicchio Radishes Rapini Salad greens (all varieties) Shallots Snow peas Spinach Sugar snap peas Sun-dried tomatoes Swiss chard Tomatoes Watercress Zucchini
SOY FOODS		
	Soy cheese Tofu	Soy cheese (low fat) Tofu (soft) Veggie breakfast links Veggie burgers

SOY FOODS

		Veggie ground round

FRESH FRUIT

Cantaloupe	Apricots	Apples
Honeydew melon	Bananas	Asian pears
Watermelon	Coconut	Avocado
	Custard apples	Blackberries
	Kiwi	Blueberries
	Mango	Cherries
	Papaya	Clementines
	Passion fruit	Cranberries
	Pineapple	Grapefruit
	Pomegranates	Grapes
		Guavas
		Lemons
		Mandarin oranges
		Nectarines
		Oranges
		Peaches
		Pears
		Plums
		Raspberries
		Rhubarb
		Strawberries
		Tangerines

NUTS		
Chocolate-covered nuts	Brazil nuts Peanuts Pecans Walnuts	Almonds Cashews Hazelnuts Macadamias Pistachios
DRIED FRUIT		
Dates Dried mango Dried papaya Dried pineapple Figs Prunes Raisins	Dried apricots Dried cranberries	Dried apples

THE DELI COUNTER

Most processed meats are high in fat, sodium and nitrates and are therefore red-light. There are, however, a few yellow- and green-light options. Cheese, too, is pretty much a diet villain, since it's high in saturated fats. However, for flavour, it can be sprinkled sparingly on salads, omelettes and pasta.

PROCESSED MEAT		
Bologna	Corned beef	Chicken breast
Hot dogs		Lean ham
Kielbasa		Pastrami (turkey)
Liverwurst		Turkey breast
Pancetta		Turkey roll
Pastrami (beef)		
Pâté		
Roast beef		
Salami		
Smoked meat		

CHEESE		
Most cheese	Low-fat cheese	Extra low-fat cheese (e.g., Laughing Cow Light, Boursin Light) Fat-free cheese
BREAD		
Flatbread	Thin whole wheat pizza crust	Whole-grain, high-fibre breads (3g fibre per slice)
OTHER		
Blue cheese dip Butternut squash dip Coleslaw Macaroni salad Polenta Tuna salad Tzatziki	Baba ghanouj	Olives Hummus Roasted red pepper dip

THE BAKERY

Anything that is made primarily of bleached white flour—which has one of the highest G.I. ratings of any food—is red-light. Because most people are in the habit of eating white bread, which has been stripped of most of its nutrients, they are unused to whole-grain breads. But once you give them a chance, I think you'll find green-light breads far more flavourful than bland white loaves.

Always check labels when choosing a loaf. The first ingredient should be 100 percent whole wheat or whole-grain flour, and there should be a minimum of 3.0 grams of fibre per slice.

While all the desserts you'll find in the bakery section are red-light because of the white flour and sugar in them, you can make your own delectable desserts at home, using the recipes in The G.I. Diet books especially the Cookbook.

BREADS		
Bagles Baguette Bread crumbs Calabrese	Crispbreads (with fibre) Pita (whole wheat)	Crispbreads (with high fibre, e.g., Wasa Fibre) Pita (high fibre)

BREADS		
Crispbreads (regular) Croissants Croutons Crumpets English muffins Hamburger buns Hot dog buns Ice cream cones Kaiser rolls Muffins Pita Raisin bread Stuffing Tortillas White bread	Tortillas (whole wheat) Whole-grain breads	Whole-grain, high-fibre breads (3g fibre per slice)

DESSERTS		
Cake Cookies Danishes Donuts Pies Tarts		

THE FISH COUNTER

All fish and shellfish are green-light and provide a wide variety of wonderful meals. Some people are under the mistaken belief that oily fish, such as salmon and mackerel, isn't good for you. In fact, oily fish is rich in omega-3 and is therefore extremely beneficial for heart health.

FISH		
All breaded fish Sushi	Fish canned in oil Salt cod	All fresh fish All frozen fish Caviar Pickled herring Sashimi Smoked fish
SHELLED FISH		
Breaded calamari Breaded clams Breaded scallops Breaded shrimp Seafood pâté	Seafood salads	Canned clams Canned crab Canned lobster Canned shrimp Fresh clams Fresh crab Imitation crab Lobster

SHELLED FISH

Mussels
Oysters
Scallops
Shrimp
Smoked oysters
Squid

THE MEAT COUNTER

Meat always contains some fat, but some cuts have far less than others. Simply trimming visible fat can reduce the overall amount by an average of 50 percent. Remember to keep the serving size to 4 ounces, which is about the size of the palm of your hand.

Skinless chicken or turkey breast is really the benchmark for low-fat protein. Dark meat, or thighs and legs, duck and goose are higher in saturated fat.

BEEF		
Brisket Regular ground beef Sausage Short ribs	Beef jerky Corned beef Lean ground beef Sirloin Sirloin tip Tenderloin	Extra-lean ground beef Eye round T-bone Top round
PORK		
Back ribs Blade Regular bacon	Centre loin Fresh ham Shank	Back bacon Lean deli ham Tenderloin

PORK		
Sausage Spareribs	Sirloin Top loin	
CHICKEN, CAPON AND TURKEY		
Breast with skin Roasters/stewing light/dark with skin Thigh with skin Wing with skin	Roasters/stewing light/dark without skin Thigh without skin Turkey bacon Turkey sausage	Breast without skin
VEAL		
Breaded cutlets Sausage		Blade steak Cutlets Loin chop Rib roast Shank
LAMB		
Rack Sausage	Fore shank Leg shank Loin chop	

DUCK AND GOOSE		
Duck (all parts) Goose (all parts)		
OTHER		
Offal Organ meat		Bison (Buffalo) Elk Emu Ostrich Rabbit Venison

THE BEANS (LEGUMES) AND CANNED VEGETABLES AISLE

Beans, or legumes, are the perfect green-light food. They are rich in protein and fibre and low in fat. Canned beans are more convenient than dried beans, but the canning process significantly raises their G.I. rating—sometimes up to 50 percent. Likewise with vegetables. It is always preferable to buy fresh or frozen vegetables rather than canned.

DRIED BEANS		
		Black beans Black-eyed peas Butter beans Chickpeas Haricots Italian Kidney beans Lentils Mung Navy Pigeon Romano Soybeans Split peas

CANNED BEANS

Baked beans with pork Broad Refried	Baked beans Chili	Baked beans (low fat) Black beans Black-eyed peas Butter beans Chickpeas Haricots Italian Lentils Mung Navy Pigeon Romano Soybeans

CANNED AND BOTTLED VEGETABLES

Artichoke hearts Creamed corn Beets Peas Potatoes Sweet potatoes Yams	Most canned vegetables Sun-dried tomatoes in oil	Canned tomatoes Roasted red peppers Tomato paste

THE PASTA AND SAUCES AISLE

Most pasta is green-light, and whole wheat pasta is even more so. Make sure to always slightly undercook pasta—until it's just *al dente*, as Italians say—and watch the serving size (6 cup cooked per serving).

Choose low-sugar pasta sauces made primarily of tomatoes. Tomato sauce happens to be rich in lycoprene, which has been shown to reduce the risk of prostate cancer. Sauces with cream and/or cheese are, of course, red-light.

PASTA		
All canned pasta		Capellini
Gnocchi		Fettuccine
Macaroni and cheese		Linguine
Noodles (canned or instant)		Macaroni
Pasta filled with cheese or meat		Penne
Rice noodles		Rigatoni
		Spaghetti
		Vermicelli

PASTA SAUCES		
Alfredo Cream sauces Sauces with added meat or cheese Sauces with added sugar or sucrose	Basil pesto Sun-dried tomato pesto	Healthy Choice pasta sauces Light sauces with vegetables (no added sugar)

THE SOUP AND CANNED SEAFOOD AND MEAT AISLE

Canned soups generally have a higher G.I. rating than soups made from scratch because of the high processing temperatures needed to prevent spoilage. So if you have the time, it's worthwhile to make your own with green-light ingredients. The best canned soups are the ones that are vegetable-based, are not puréed and don't contain cream.

SOUP		
All cream-based soups Canned black bean Canned green pea Canned puréed vegetable Canned split pea Instant soups	Canned chicken noodle Canned lentil Canned tomato	Campbells' Healthy Request soups Canned low-fat bean and vegetable soups Miso soup
CANNED SEAFOOD		
	Fish canned in oil	Fish canned in water Shrimp Smoked oysters

CANNED MEAT

Beef	Chicken	
Ham	Turkey	
Pork		
Spam		

THE GRAINS AND SIDE DISHES AISLE

Whole grains with all the nutrition and fibre intact are usually green-light. With rice, it all depends on the variety, because some contain a starch, amylase, that breaks down more slowly.

GRAINS		
Arborio rice	Cornmeal	Barley
Couscous	Kamut	Basmati rice
Grits	Spelt	Brown rice
Instant rice	Whole wheat couscous	Buckwheat
Jasmine rice		Bulgar
Millet		Graham
Semolina		Flax seeds
Short-grain rice		Kasha
Sticky rice		Long-grain rice
		Quinoa
		Wheat berries
		Wild rice
SIDE DISHES		
Instant noodles		
Instant potatoes		
Stuffing		

THE INTERNATIONAL FOODS AISLE

Choosing the right oil to use in cooking and on salads is critical to your heart health. Saturated and hydrogenated oils are dangerous and should be avoided. Canola and olive oils get the green light.

Because acid tends to reduce the G.I. rating of a meal—it slows the digestive process—vinegars and vinaigrettes are great additions. Dressings should always be low-fat, but be careful of sugar levels. Sometimes producers will raise the sugar level as they reduce the oil to improve flavour. Be sure to check labels and compare low-fat brands.

ASIAN		
Canned lychees in syrup	Black bean sauce	Buckwheat noodles
Chow mein noodles	Canned baby corn	Canned bamboo shoots
Chutney	Canned lychees in juice	Canned water chestnuts
Coconut milk	Chili-garlic sauce	Cellophane (mung bean) noodles
Ghee	Coconut milk (light)	Curry paste
Honey garlic sauce	Fish sauce	Dried seaweed
Instant noodles	Oyster sauce	Hoisin sauce
Plum sauce	Pappadums (baked)	Hot chili paste
Ramen noodles		

ASIAN		
Rice noodles Sweet and sour sauce	Rice wine Sesame oil Soy sauce (regular) Udon noodles	Miso Pickled ginger Rice vinegar Soy sauce (low sodium) Teriyaki sauce Vermicelli Wasabi
MEXICAN		
Refried beans Taco shells Tortillas Tostados	Salsa (with added sugar) Taco sauce (with added sugar)	Canned green chiles Chipotle en adobo Pickled jalapenos Salsa (with no added sugar) Taco sauce (with no added sugar)
MIDDLE EASTERN		
Couscous Pita bread Stuffed grape leaves	Baba ghanouj Whole wheat pita bread	Falafel mix Hummus Tahini

THE COOKING OIL, VINEGAR, SALAD DRESSING AND PICKLES AISLE

Choosing the right oil to use in cooking and on salads is critical to your heart health. Saturated and hydrogenated oils are dangerous and should be avoided. Canola and olive oils get the green light.

Because acid tends to reduce the G.I. rating of a meal—it slows the digestive process—vinegars and vinaigrettes are great additions. Dressings should always be low-fat, but be careful of sugar levels. Sometimes producers will raise the sugar level as they reduce the oil to improve flavour. Be sure to check labels and compare low-fat brands.

COOKING OIL		
Coconut oil Palm oil Vegetable shortening	Corn oil Peanut oil Sesame oil Soybean oil Sunflower oil Vegetable oil	Canola oil Extra-virgin olive oil Flax oil Olive oil Vegetable oil spray

VINEGAR		
		Balsamic vinegar Cider vinegar Red wine vinegar Red wine vinegar Rice vinegar White vinegar White wine vinegar
SALAD DRESSINGS		
Regular salad dressings	Light salad dressings	Low-fat, low sugar salad dressings Low-fat, low sugar vinaigrettes
PICKLES		
Branston pickle Bread and butter pickles Chow chow Chutney Gherkins Pickled beets	Sun-dried tomatoes in oil	Capers Cocktail onions Dill pickles Olives Pickled hot peppers Pickled mixed vegetables

PICKLES		
Sweet mustard pickles		Pickled mushrooms Sauerkraut
CONDIMENTS		
Barbecue sauce Chili sauce Honey mustard Ketchup Mayonnaise Relish Steak sauce Tartar sauce	Hot sauce Salsa (with added sugar)	Dijon mustard Gravy mix (maximum 20 calories per ¼ cup serving) Horseradish Hummus Mayonnaise (fat free) Mustard Salsa (no added sugar) Sauerkraut Seafood cocktail sauce Soy sauce (low sodium) Tabasco Vinegar Worcestershire sauce

THE SNACKS AISLE

Unfortunately, the snacks aisle at the supermarket is full of red-light temptation. Still, all you G.I. Dieters need three snacks a day—green-light ones of course. If you purchase food bars, make sure they contain most importantly 12 to 15 grams of protein per 50 g bar. Good green-light choices are Balance and Zone bars (half a bar per serving).

SNACKS		
Candy Caramel-coated popcorn Cheesies Crackers Crispbreads (regular) Flavoured gelatin (all varieties) Fruit leather Granola bars Ice cream cones Melba toast Party mix Popcorn (regular) Potato chips	Crispbreads (with fibre) Dark chocolate (70% cocoa) Most nuts Popcorn (air-popped) Roasted peanuts Salsa (with added sugar)	Almonds Applesauce (unsweetened) Canned fruit salad Canned mandarin oranges Canned peaches in juice or water Canned pears in juice or water Cashews Crispbreads with high fibre, e.g., Wasa Fibre)

SNACKS		
Pretzels Pudding Raisins Rice cakes Rice chips Rice crackers Tortilla chips Trail mix		Food bars Fruit bowls with no added sugar Hazelnuts Macadamia nuts Pistachios Pumpkin seeds Salsa (with no added sugar) Soynuts Sugar-free hard candies Sunflower seeds

THE BAKING AISLE

Though you can't eat ready-made baked goods from the supermarket when you're trying to lose weight, you can bake your own sweet treats using recipes from the G.I. Diet books. They call for sugar substitutes rather than sugar, honey or molasses. Our favourite brand of sweetener is Splenda, which is derived from sugar but doesn't have the calories. It measures by volume exactly as sugar does. Although dried fruit such as raisins and cranberries are red- and yellow-light, small amounts are acceptable for baking.

SWEETENERS		
Agave nectar Corn syrup Glucose Honey Molasses Splenda Brown Sugar (all types)	Fructose Sugar alcohols	Brown sugar substitute (e.g., Sugar Twin Brown) Splenda Stevia (note: not FDA approved) Sugar Twin Sweet 'N Low

BAKING SUPPLIES

- Cake mixes
- Canned cranberry sauce
- Canned pumpkin
- Chocolate chips
- Cookie mixes
- Evaporated milk
- Glacé cherries
- Graham cracker crumbs
- Icing
- Lard
- Maraschino cherries
- Mincemeat
- Muffin mixes
- Peanut butter (regular and light)
- Pie filling
- Prunes
- Raisins
- Sweetened condensed milk
- Vegetable shortening
- White flour

- 100% nut butters
- 100% peanut butter
- Baking chocolate (unsweetened)
- Coconut
- Dried apricots
- Dried cranberries
- Peanuts
- Pecans
- Pine nuts
- Walnuts

- Almonds
- Baking powder
- Baking soda
- Cashews
- Cocoa
- Hazelnuts
- Macadamia nuts
- Oat bran
- Pumpkin seeds
- Sunflower seeds
- Wheat bran
- Wheat germ
- Whole wheat flour

SPICES AND FLAVOURINGS		
Coating for poultry or pork	Bouillon Bovril Marmite	Bouillon (low sodium) Chili powder Dried herbs Extracts (vanilla, etc.) Garlic Gravy mixes (20 calories maximum per ¼ cup serving) Lemon juice Lime juice Pepper Salt Seasoning mixes with no added sugar Spices

THE BREAKFAST FOODS AISLE

Of course, the king of breakfast foods is old-fashioned oatmeal—the large-flake kind, not instant or quick oats. Most cereals on the market are red-light. They are made from highly processed grains that lack both nutrition and fibre. Beware of those so-called healthy or natural granola types of cereal, because they, too, are usually low in fibre and high in sugar. What you should be looking for are cereals that have at least 10 grams of fibre per serving. While they may not seem much fun in themselves, they can be dressed up with nuts, fruit and yogurt. Cereal bars are absolutely red-light—they're full of sugar. Better to go for a Balance or Zone bar or equivalent.

While packaged pancake mixes and frozen waffles are red-light, you can make green-light versions yourself (the recipes are in *The G.I. Diet Cookbook*). Low-sugar fruit spreads that list fruit as the first ingredient are wonderful green-light additions to toast, cereal and low-fat dairy products, such as yogurt and cottage cheese.

CEREALS

All cold cereals except those listed as yellow or red light	Kashi Good Friends	100% Bran
Cereal bars	Shredded Wheat Bran	All-Bran
Cream of wheat		Bran Buds
Granola		Fibre 1
Instant porridge		Fibre First
Muesli		Kashi Go Lean
Quick-cooking oatmeal		Kashi Go Lean Crunch
		Large-flake oatmeal
		Oat bran
		Red River
		Steel-cut oatmeal

PANCAKES AND SYRUPS

Corn syrup		
Maple syrup		
Molasses		
Pancake mix		
Pancake syrup		

SPREADS

Fruit spreads (regular)	100% nut butters	Fruit spreads (extra fruit, no added sugar)
Jam	100% peanut butter	

SPREADS		
Marmalade Nutella Peanut butter (regular and light)		

THE BEVERAGE AISLE

You need up to eight glasses of liquid a day to keep your body hydrated and healthy. Drinks with caffeine tend to stimulate the appetite and so are red-light. The exception is tea, which has far less caffeine than either coffee or soft drinks. Juice is not worth the extra calories—eat the fruit instead. In addition to the green-light beverages listed below, remember that skim milk and light plain soy milk, which are found in the dairy section, also make refreshing and nutritious drinks.

BEVERAGES		
Chocolate milk mix	Diet soft drinks (caffeinated)	Bottled water (carbonated or non-carbonated)
Coffee whitener	Most unsweetened juice	Club soda
Evaporated milk	Non-alcoholic beer	Decaffeinated coffee
Fruit crystals	Vegetable juices	Diet soft drinks (without caffeine)
Fruit drinks		Herbal teas
Hot chocolate (regular)		Hot chocolate (light)
Regular coffee		
Regular iced tea		
Regualr soft drinks		
Sports drinks		

BEVERAGES		
Sweetened condensed milk Sweetened juice Watermelon juice		Iced tea (with no added sugar) Tea (with or without caffeine)

THE DAIRY CASE

Low-fat dairy products are a G.I. Diet staple. They are rich in protein, calcium and vitamin D. Regular dairy products contain a high amount of saturated fat and are therefore red-light. But you can lightly sprinkle full-flavoured cheeses such as old cheddar, feta and Parmesan over salads, omelettes and pasta. If you are lactose intolerant, low-fat soy products are an excellent alternative—just make sure they aren't laden with sugar.

There is a wide selection of non-dairy products in the dairy case, such as pickles, cookie dough and anchovy paste. I've listed some of these items too.

MILK		
Almond milk Chocolate milk Cream Goat milk Regular soy milk Rice milk Whole or 2% milk	1% milk Coconut milk (low-fat)	Buttermilk Skim milk Soy milk (plain, low-fat)

CHEESE		
Cheese (regular) Cheese spread Cottage cheese (whole or 2%) Cream cheese	Cheese (low-fat) Low-fat cream cheese Low-fat string cheese Regular soy cheese	Cheese (fat-free) Cottage cheese (1% or fat-free) Extra low-fat cheese (e.g., Laughing Cow Light, Boursin Light) Low-fat soy cheese
YOGURT AND SOUR CREAM		
Sour cream Yogurt (whole or 2%)	Sour cream (light) Yogurt (low-fat with sugar)	Fruit yogurt (nonfat with sweetener) Sour cream (nonfat)
BUTTER AND MARGARINE		
Butter Hard margarine	Soft margarine (non-hydrogenated)	Soft margarine (non-dydrogenated, light)

EGGS		
	Whole regular eggs (preferably omega-3)	Egg whites in cartons Liquid eggs in cartons Naturegg Break Free Naturegg Omega Pro

OTHER		
Bread and butter pickles Eggnog Cookie dough Dips Flavoured gelatin Pickled eggs Pudding Sweetened juice	Anchovy paste Unsweetened juice	Dill pickles Gefilte fish Horseradish Pickled herring Pickled sweet pimentos Pickled tomatoes

THE FROZEN FOOD SECTION

Almost all of the prepared meals you find in the frozen food section of your grocery store are red-light because of the ingredients used and the way in which they've been processed. Still, the freezer section is a great source for green-light convenience foods such as frozen vegetables and fruit, fish and green-light desserts. Make sure the vegetables aren't in a butter, cream or cheese sauce—that's definitely red-light!

VEGETABLES		
Broad beans	Artichoke hearts	Asparagus
French fries	Corn	Beans (green/ wax)
Hash browns	Squash	Bell peppers
Lima beans		Broccoli
Rutabaga		Brussels sprouts
Vegetables in a butter, cream or cheese sauce		Carrots
		Cauliflower
		Fiddleheads
		Okra
		Peas
		Spinach

PREPARED FOOD		
Appetizers Chicken wings Dumplings Lasagna Meat pies Pasta filled with cheese or meat Perogies Pizza Rice dishes TV dinners White bread	Lean burgers Pork souvlaki Turkey burgers	Chicken souvlaki Extra-lean burgers Frozen fish without breaded coating Scallops without breaded coating Shrimp without breaded coating Veggie burgers Veggie ground round
BREAKFAST		
Hash browns Sausages Waffles		Egg Beaters Veggie breakfast links

DESSERTS		
Frozen soy desserts (regular) Ice cream (regular) Pie Pie and tart shells Popsicles Puff pastry Tartufo Whipped topping	Fruit bars (no added sugar)	Frozen soy desserts with about 100 calories or less per ¼ cup Frozen yogurt (low-fat) Ice cream (low-fat and no sugar added)
FRUIT		
		Blackberries Blueberries Cherries Cranberries Peaches Raspberries Rhubarb Strawberries

PART TWO

Eating Out

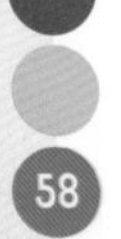

The Green-Light Fast Food Guide

Just a few years ago, the idea of ordering a green-light lunch at a fast food outlet was simply laughable—but no longer! Due in part to the threat of legal action and in part to stagnant market shares, the major fast food chains are finally offering some healthy options. In all fairness, Subway has been pioneering the move toward fast, healthy meals for some time now, and their initiative has been reflected in their phenomenal growth. They have actually replaced McDonald's as North America's number one fast food chain.

Unfortunately, the majority of the food on offer at fast food restaurants is still red-light: hamburgers soaked in saturated fat, fish and chicken coated in deep-fried batter, and all the trimmings, such as fries, sodas, shakes and ketchup, loaded with fat and sugar. To compound this dietary disaster, you can supersize everything! No wonder we're setting obesity records and becoming diabetics at an exponential rate.

So, what are the points of light in this sea of gloom? I've listed them by each major fast food chain. **Remember to always discard the top half of the bun on burgers or sandwiches and eat them open-faced; and to ask for low-fat dressings and use only one third of the sachet on your salad.** You can just about swim in a full sachet. **Also, always choose grilled, not fried, (crispy) chicken.**

One of the health issues that is rarely mentioned in the de bate on fast food is sodium levels. When creating lower fat products, the fast food industry frequently boosts salt content to make up for any perceived flavour shortfall. The problem is that sodium increases water retention, which causes bloating and extra weight—especially in women—and raises blood pressure. The official recommended daily allowance of sodium is 2,500 milligrams, but the leading authorities are calling for a reduction to 1,500 milligrams. On average we consume more than twice that. Though Swiss Chalet's Grilled Chicken

Breast on Rice appears to be a healthy, low-fat meal, it contains 2,420 milligrams of sodium, or nearly twice what you need for an entire day! In order to alert you to the sodium levels in the fast food I've listed, **I've asterixed those items that have excessively high levels.**

Though I've done my best to ensure that the information is the latest available at time of printing, this is a rapidly changing field. You might want to check the website of your favorite fast foods outlet from time to time.

McDONALD'S

SALADS

Spicy Thai Chicken Salad with *grilled* chicken [not crispy]
Garden Fresh Salad with *grilled* chicken
Mediterranean Salad with *grilled* chicken*

DRESSINGS

Renee's Ravin' Raspberry Vinaigrette

OTHER MEALS

Chicken fajita
Spicy Buffalo Grilled Chicken Snack

SNACK

Fruit 'n Yogurt Parfait (hold the granola)
Apple Slices with caramel dip

WENDY'S

SALADS

Mandarin Chicken Salad [hold the noodles]
Chicken Caesar Salad [hold croutons; use dressing below]

DRESSINGS

Balsamic Vinaigrette
Light Classic Ranch
Light Honey Dijon

BURGERS/WRAPS

Ultimate Chicken Grill* plus side salad
Grilled Chicken Go Wrap

CHILI

Large chili plus side salad

SNACK

Jr. Frosty Dairy Dessert (6 oz cup)

BURGER KING

Unfortunately this chain is one of the few that does not appear to have got the message that people want healthy options.

SALADS

Salads are loaded with fat and sodium. Stay clear.

BURGERS

BK VEGGIE* plus side salad

HARVEY'S

SALADS

Entrée Grilled Chicken Garden Salad

DRESSINGS

Asian Sesame

Light Italian

BURGERS

Signature Grilled Chicken*

Veggieburger

SUBWAY

The best choice of roll for a sub is 9 Grain Wheat or Honey Oat.

SUBS (6-INCH) OR FLATBREAD

Roast Beef
Oven Roasted Chicken Breast
Turkey Breast*
Veggie Delite

SALADS

Ham
Chicken
Beef
Chicken teriyaki
Turkey breast and ham
Veggie delite

DRESSING

Fat Free Italian

SOUP

Chicken Tortilla

TIM HORTONS

This chain has a major problem with high sodium. For instance their Turkey Bacon Club sandwich and mushroom soup deliver nearly twice the recommended total daily consumption of salt. There are a few acceptable choices.

SANDWICHES

Toasted chicken club
Chicken salad

SOUPS

Chicken noodle*
Minestrone*

SWISS CHALET

MEALS

Classic Quarter Chicken (white meat skinless)
Chicken on a Kaiser (white meat skinless)
Hot Chicken Sandwich (white meat skinless)

SIDES

Greek salad
Garden salad
Fresh vegetable medley

SALADS

Spinach Chicken Salad (hold the tortilla)

DRESSINGS

Light Italian
Fat-Free Raspberry Vinaigrette

DESSERT

Cranberry Raspberry Frozen Yogurt

PIZZA HUT

PIZZA

Only selecte the **Thin 'n Crispy** version of the following pizzas. Maximum serving two slices.

Chicken Lovers Deluxe
Chicken Caesar Pizza
Chicken Italiano
Greek
Veggie Lovers

SALADS

Greek
Garden

DRESSING

Honey mustard

TACO BELL

TACO

Fresno beef hard taco
Fresno beef soft taco
Fresno grilled steak soft taco
Fresno grilled chicken soft taco
Fresno spicy chicken soft taco

KFC

Until KFC adopts grilled, as opposed to fried chicken as they have in the US, it's a place to avoid.

* Limit foods with excessively high levels of sodium.

The Green-Light Restaurant Guide

It isn't difficult to dine out the green-light way now that restaurants are following healthy trends such as broiling and grilling instead of frying, using vegetable oils and offering a greater variety of fish dishes, vegetables and salads. Here are my top ten tips for ensuring your night out doesn't leave you feeling guilty the next day:

1. If possible, eat a small bowl of green-light cereal with skim milk and sweetener just before you leave for the restaurant. This will give you some extra fibre and help take the edge off your appetite.

2. On arrival at the restaurant, drink a glass of water to help you feel a bit fuller. Feel free to enjoy a glass of red wine, but wait until the main course arrives to drink it.

3. Once the habitual basket of rolls or bread—which you ignore—has been passed around the table, ask the waiter to remove it. The longer it sits there, the more tempted you'll be to dig in.

4. Order a chunky vegetable-based soup or a salad with the dressing on the side (no Caesar) to start with, and tell your waiter you'd like this as soon as possible.

5. Ask for vegetables instead of potatoes and rice, since you can't be sure what type will be served.

6. Stick with low-fat cuts of meat or poultry (see page 22–24), or choose fish or shellfish that isn't breaded or battered. Because restaurant servings tend to be overly generous, remember to eat only 4 to 6 ounces (about the size of a pack of cards) and leave the rest.

7. Ask that any sauces that come with your meal be put on the side.

8. Desserts are almost always a dietary minefield with not a lot of green-light choices. Fresh fruit or

berries without ice cream is the best option. Or perhaps order a decaffeinated skim-milk latte and sweeten it with sugar substitute.

If social pressure to have a rich dessert becomes overwhelming, ask for extra forks so it can be shared. A couple of forkfuls or so with your coffee should get you off the hook with minimal dietary damage!

9. Order only decaffeinated coffee or tea. My favourite choice is a nonfat decaf cappuccino.

10. Finally, and perhaps most importantly, eat slowly. The famous Dr. Johnson advised chewing food thirty-two times before swallowing! Although that is a bit over the top, at least try to put your fork down between mouthfuls. The stomach can take between 20 and 30 minutes to let the brain know it's full.

Because of the local nature of most of the restaurant industry, it is impossible for me to make specific recommendations for specific restaurants. Accordingly, I have grouped restaurants into 10 principal categories and made recommendations as what to choose and what to avoid.

FAMILY RESTAURANTS

This is a fast growing segment of the restaurant business and offers a very wide choice of foods and good value for a family eating out.

Though there are a few national chains, such as Kelsey's, most are local operations. It would therefore be physically impossible to break out individual restaurants in the space available.

However, the one overriding caution with these restaurants is portion size. Many serving sizes are large enough for two people. On a recent road trip, my wife and I found we could split many, if not most, of the courses and still come away satisfied.

If you are watchful, you can easily find many green-light alternatives to suit all the family.

ALL-YOU-CAN-EAT BUFFETS

A buffet can be your best or worst option, depending on your level of self-control. While you're free to make your own selections, there may be a lot of red-light temptations there. I suggest you do a quick reconnaissance of the whole buffet before picking up your plate and starting in. This will ensure there's still space on your plate when you reach your favourite foods. Follow the G.I. Diet ground rules, and the buffet will be your best dining-out option bar none.

INTERNATIONAL CUISINE

When eating the same type of food week after week starts to get a bit uninspiring, how about trying something completely new? I love international cuisine, particularly Italian, Greek, Chinese and Indian food. Because we're often unfamiliar with how an exotic dish is made, it's hard to determine whether it's green light or not. In this section I've tried to eliminate some of the guesswork by listing the dishes you'd typically find on a menu. Don't hesitate to ask your server about any dish I haven't mentioned. Here's a list of possible questions that could help give your meal a green light:

- Is this food fried, grilled or steamed?
- Could you ask the chef to prepare this dish without the cream sauce?

- Could the chef prepare this dish with the least amount of oil possible?
- Could I order only a half serving of this dish?
- Could you replace the potatoes with extra vegetables?
- Could I have the dressing/gravy/sauce on the side?

ITALIAN

If you're serious about sticking to the G.I. Diet, it's really not a good idea to head to a pizzeria. Instead, go to a restaurant that has a wide variety of dishes on the menu. Usually these are divided into a number of parts: L'antipasto, which translates as "before the meal," includes hot and cold appetizers; il primo, or "the first course," includes pasta, pizza or risotto; il secondo, "the second course," includes meat, poultry or fish; and il dolce is "dessert."

Your best bets on the list of antipasti are soups containing beans and vegetables, such as minestrone, and salads, particularly the basic insalata mista. Remember to ask for the dressing on the side. Mussels are a good choice provided they are not served in a cream sauce. Other antipasto items such as roasted red peppers or mushrooms sound both delicious and healthy, but be careful of any that are marinated in oil. Although olive oil is beneficial, it is still calorie-dense. One cup equals the total daily calorie requirement for most people.

Although you should never make a meal of pasta, you can enjoy it as a first course. Choose pasta with a tomato-based sauce and share it with a dinner companion. Your serving should not exceed one quarter of the plate. Avoid pasta stuffed with meat and cheese, pasta in cream sauces and gnocchi. Decline the offer of grated cheese.

If you're craving pizza instead of pasta, choose one with a very thin crust, tomato sauce and vegetable toppings. Ask for no cheese except for a sprinkling of Parmesan. Then have only one slice, sharing the rest with the others at the table. Pizza should also be treated as an appetizer rather than as a meal.

For your secondo, choose grilled, roasted or braised fish, chicken or meat. Veal, a mainstay on Italian menus, is low in saturated fat and therefore an excellent choice, unless it is cooked in butter or served with cream sauce. Watch the serving size—you can always leave some on your plate if necessary. The Italian restaurant I frequent serves a fabulous veal chop, but it is about 14 ounces and comes with mashed potatoes. I ask for extra vegetables instead of the potatoes and share the veal with my wife, Ruth. We also order an extra vegetable or pasta dish to share.

For dessert I highly recommend a skim-milk decaf cappuccino—delicious! You won't miss the highly fattening tiramisu. If you're in a celebratory mood, treat yourself to some gelato, but since it is high in sugar, split it with a friend.

ITALIAN		
Breaded eggplant (or any breaded vegetable) Fried calamari Garlic bread Gnocchi Mozzarella or bocconcini and tomato salads Pasta filled with meat or cheese Pasta with cream or cheese sauce Risotto Salads with creamy dressings such as Caesar	Mussels in wine sauce (no cream) Roasted or braised lamb (loin/leg) Thin-crust pizzas without cheese	Grilled fish and chicken Grilled shrimp, scallops or calamari Grilled, steamed or boiled vegetables Mussels with tomato sauce 9no wine) Pasta with seafood in tomato sauce(¼ plate only) Pasta with vegetables in tomato sauce (¼ plate only) Roasted fish Veal without cream or butter sauce

GREEK

Greek restaurants often offer a selection of small dishes called meze. Two or three of these, such as hummus and grilled calamari can be a meal in themselves when served with small pieces of whole wheat pita and raw vegetables for dipping.

Grilled or baked seafood makes an excellent dinner choice. And the classic chicken souvlaki dinner can also be good. Though the serving sizes are often too large, just stick to the recommended green-light servings and you'll be fine. If the rice appears glutinous or sticky avoid it. If potatoes are served with the rice, ask for vegetables instead. A Greek salad often comes with your souvlaki dinner. If this is the case, ask that the feta and dressing be served on the side.

Greek desserts are calorie-laden—particularly the ever-popular baklava—and thus red-light.

GREEK

Baklava	Baba ghanouj	Chicken souvlaki
Breaded calamari	Grilled lamb chops	Grilled or baked seafood
Dolmades	Grilled loin lamb chops	Hummus
Gyros	Lamb souvlaki	Melitzanosalata
Kleftiko	Pork souvlaki	
Moussaka	Vegetable gemistes	
Pastitsio		
Potato gemistes		
Spanakopita (spinach pie)		
Tzatziki		

CHINESE

It's a real challenge to eat the green-light way at a Chinese restaurant. Much of the food is deep-fried or drowning in sweet sauces and therefore a disaster for your waistline. The sodium levels in the sauces are often very high, and saturated and trans fat oils are sometimes used in cooking. However it is not impossible to get a green-light meal. Pass on the spring rolls, crispy fried duck, fried rice and dumplings, and look for dishes that contain steamed or stir-fried vegetables with oyster sauce, garlic and ginger. Since many Chinese dishes rest on beds of rice or noodles, you need to pay attention to both type and amount. Most of the rice used is short grain with a glutinous sticky surface, and this is red-light. Ask if they have long grain or brown rice instead—you may be lucky. Make sure it is steamed.

Noodles, for the most part, are red-light, except for "cellophane noodles," which are made from mung beans. Keep the noodle proportion to no more than one quarter of your plate—it's too easy to heap them up. Stick with savoury sauces and avoid sweet and sour dishes. Try eating with

chopsticks—they will slow you down so you end up eating less.

CHINESE		
Chinese omelettes Chow mein Dumplings Lo mein Spring rolls Sweet and sour dishes Wonton soup	Beef in black bean sauce Egg noodles Stir-fried seafood, chicken or meat with vegetables (cooked in a small amount of oil)	Cellophane noodles (mung bean noodles) Hot and sour soup Sautéed vegetables with garlic Steamed seafood Steamed tofu with vegetables Steamed vegetables

INDIAN/SOUTH ASIAN

Vegetables, legumes and basmati rice are predominant in Indian cuisine. Many South Asians are vegetarians whose protein source is lentils and beans. Servings of meat, poultry or fish tend to be modest when used, and all this makes an Indian restaurant an excellent green-light dining option.

There are, however a few problems to watch for. The first is that the food is often fried. To make things worse, the food is often fried in "ghee," or clarified butter, a highly saturated fat. Be sure to ask your server how the food is prepared. Choose dishes that are baked or broiled.

The second problem is that full-fat dairy products are sometimes used. Try to avoid dishes with creamy sauces. And avoid the bread, which is often made with ghee. If you really, really want bread, choose baked whole wheat chapati. But it is better to have basmati rice instead. Don't have both.

Many restaurants offer their patrons heaped dishes of coconut slices, raisins and other sweeteners. These are red-light. Similarly be careful of the addition of mangoes and papayas, which are yellow-light, in dishes. Guavas are green-light.

INDIAN		
Butter chicken	Baked chapatti	Balti vegetables
Chicken biryani	Prawns madras	Bengan bharta
Chicken korma		Chicken or fish saag
Chicken tikka masala		Chicken tikka
Curries with cream sauces		Chicken tikka kebab
Lamb rogan josh		Chicken vindaloo
Naan		Dal
Pakoras		Fish kebab
		Grilled fish
		Lentil or bean dishes without cream sauces
		Steamed basmati rice
		Tandoori chicken or fish
		Vegetable curries without cream sauces

MEXICAN/LATIN AMERICAN

Tex-Mex dishes that are heavy on cheese, refried beans, sour cream and tortillas are unsurprisingly red light. Most "blackened" dishes are pan-fried in garlic butter, and so must be avoided as well. Look for grilled seafood, chicken or meat with salsa, or dishes made with beans (not refried). Gazpacho soups made with tomatoes and peppers are excellent, as is ceviche, which is a seafood dish prepared with citrus juices.

MEXICAN		
Burritos Chorizo Nachos Quesadillas	Chicken fjitas without the cheese and sour cream Chicken or vegetable enchiladas with red sauce or salsa Chili with meat and beans	Arroz a banda (fish with rice) Baked fish Bean and vegetable soups Ceviche Chili with beans Chili with chicken and beans Gazpacho Grilled fish

THAI

Green-light eating is a challenge in Thai restaurants. In North America they tend to rely on sauces to create flavour, rather than spices and herbs as they do in Thailand. Many sauces are very sweet: tamarind sauce, Thai basil sauce and oyster sauce are all red-light. Pad Thai, probably the most popular dish, is made with tamarind sauce and rice noodles. Curry sauces and peanut sauce are usually made with full-fat coconut milk and should be avoided, too. "Gee," you must be thinking, "is there anything I *can* eat in a Thai restaurant?"

The answer is yes. Start with a lemongrass broth. Then have a Thai beef salad, or a stir-fry with chicken and vegetables. Many Thai stir-fries are cooked quickly in small amounts of oil. Satays are also an excellent choice, but skip the peanut sauce. Have your satay with stir-fried or steamed vegetables and a green mango or papaya salad for a fabulous meal.

THAI		
Curries containing coconut milk Fried rice noodles Fried spring rolls Pad Thai Soups containing coconut milk	Cold rolls (watch the dips) Green mango salad (dressing on the side) Papaya salad	Chicken or beef satays Hot and sour soup Seafood or vegetable soup without coconut milk Steamed seafood Thai beef or chicken salad (dressing on the side) Vegetables stir-fried with little oil

JAPANESE

There are lots of wonderful green-light options at Japanese restaurants once you get beyond the sushi and tempura. Sushi is red-light because of the glutinous rice it is made with. Order sashimi instead, which is the fish without the rice. Watch the quantity of soy sauce you use—it's very high in sodium and should be thought of as liquid salt. Other Japanese specialties include wonderful soups made with clear broth bases, sukiyaki, which is a beef and vegetable stir-fry that uses a minimal amount of vegetable oil, and grilled fish. In many restaurants you can prepare your meal yourself in your own group pot. Nabemono is like a healthy fondue. Into the pot of boiling broth go chunks of vegetables, seafood and so on. Not only is it delicious, but it's a fun experience to share with friends. Miso soup is an excellent source of protein, and in Japan it is eaten at the end of the meal to aid digestion.

JAPANESE		
Agemono (deep-freid) Beef teriyaki Deep-fried pork dishes Gyoza (fired dumplings) Oyako-donburi (chicken omelette over rice) Sushi Tempura	Chicken teriyaki Noodle soups Pickled salads Shabu-shabu Udon	Grilled seafood Miso soup Nabemono (seafood and vegetables in a broth) Sashimi Soba Steamed rice and vegetables Stir-fried vegetables Sukiyaki Sumashi wan (clear soup with tofu and shrimp) Yosenabe (casseroles)

INDEX

Rick Gallop's bestselling *G.I. Diet* was published in 2002 and quickly became the most successful Canadian diet book ever, with more than two million copies sold worldwide. It is currently available in twenty-three countries, in a dozen different languages. Gallop holds a Masters degree from Oxford University and was president and CEO of the Heart and Stroke Foundation of Ontario.